The Definitive Air Fryer Cookbook

A Handful of Quick, Delicious Recipes for Your Air Fryer Meals

Kira Hamm

TABLE OF CONTENT

Orange Sauce with Trout Fillet

Preparation Time 10 minutes

Cooking Time:10 minutes

Servings: 5

Ingredients:

- 1 tbsp of minced ginger
- 5 chopped spring onion
- Black pepper and salt
- 1 orange juice and zest
- 1 tbsp of olive oil
- 5 trout fillets

Directions:

1. Sprinkle pepper and salt over the trout fillet.
2. Brush the fillets with olive oil.
3. Transfer the fillets to the Power XL Air Fryer Grill pan.
4. Add spring onion, orange juice and zest, and ginger to the grill pan.
5. Set the Power XL Air Fryer Grill to Air fryer/Grill.
6. Grill for about 10 minutes at 3600F.

7. Serve immediately

8. Serving Suggestions: Serve with the orange sauce

9. Directions: & Cooking Tips: remove the skin and bone of the trout fillets

Nutrition: Calories: 348kcal, Fat: 14g, Carb: 15g, Proteins: 42g

Grilled Parsley and Thyme Salmon

Preparation Time 10 minutes

Cooking Time:10 minutes

Servings: 5

Ingredients:

- 5 parsley sprigs
- 5 salmon fillets
- 1 chopped yellow onion
- 3 tbsp of olive oil
- 3 sliced tomatoes
- 5 thyme sprigs
- Black pepper and salt
- 1 lemon juice

Directions:

1. Pour 1 tbsp of oil on the Power XL Air Fryer Grill pan.
2. Add the sliced tomatoes to the grill pan.
3. Sprinkle pepper and salt on the tomatoes.
4. Pour another 1 tbsp of oil on the grill pan.
5. Place onion, fish, parsley spring, lemon juice, thyme sprig on the tomatoes.

6. Transfer the pan to the Power XL Air Fryer Grill basket

7. Set the Power XL Air Fryer Grill to Air fryer/Grill.

8. Set the Timer to 12 minutes and temperature at 3600F

9. Serve immediately

10. Serving Suggestions: Serve with your favorite sauce

11. Directions: & Cooking Tips: Debone the fillets

Nutrition: Calories: 290kcal, Fat: 10g, Carb: 15g, Proteins: 32g

Grilled Mustard Salmon

Preparation Time: 15 minutes

Cooking Time: 10 minutes

Serving: 2

Ingredients:

- 1 tbsp of coconut oil
- 2 large salmon fillets
- 2 tbsp of mustard
- 1 tbsp of maple extract
- Black pepper and salt

Directions:

1. Mix mustard, salmon, maple extract, pepper, and salt in a bowl.
2. Drizzle the fish with cooking oil.
3. Place the fish on the Power XL Air Fryer Grill basket at position 6.
4. Set the Power XL Air Fryer Grill to Air fryer/Grill.
5. Set the Timer to 10 minutes at 3700F.
6. Serve immediately.
7. Serving Suggestions: remove the salmon bone before cooking.

8. Directions: & Cooking Tips: Serve with maple syrup

Nutrition: Calories: 300kcal, Fat: 22g, Carb: 2.5g, Proteins: 25g

Tabasco Shrimps

Preparation Time: 15 minutes

Cooking Time: 10 minutes

Servings: 5

Ingredients:

- 1 tsp of oregano
- Black pepper and pepper
- 1 pound of shrimp
- 1/2 tsp of smoked paprika
- 1 tsp of Tabasco sauce
- 1 tsp of red pepper flakes
- 1/2 tsp of parsley
- 2 tbsp of olive oil
- 2 tbsp of water

Directions:

1. Mix shrimps, pepper, salt, and water in a bowl.
2. Add pepper flakes, parsley, paprika, tabasco sauce, and oregano.
3. Mix well
4. Preheat the Power XL Air Fryer Grill.
5. Place the mixture on the Power XL Air Fryer Grill basket.

6. Set the Power XL Air Fryer Grill to Air fryer/Grill.

7. Grill for 10 minutes at 3700F.

8. Serving Suggestions: serve with salad

9. Directions: & Cooking Tips: rinse shrimp well before coating

Nutrition: Calories: 210kcal, Fat: 13g, Carb: 2g, Proteins: 22g

Buttered Shrimps

Preparation time 10 minutes

Cooking Time:6 minutes

Servings: 3

Ingredients:

- 1 tbsp of chopped rosemary
- Black pepper and salt
- 10 shrimps
- 10 slices of green bell pepper
- 4 cloves of garlic
- 1 tbsp of melted butter

Directions:

1. Mix butter, rosemary, shrimps, and pepper in a bowl.
2. Add garlic, bell pepper, and salt.
3. Allow to rest for 5 minutes.
4. Place the shrimp mix on the Power XL Air Fryer Grill basket.
5. Set the Power XL Air Fryer Grill to Air fryer/Grill.
6. Leave to grill for about 6 minutes at 3600F.
7. Serve immediately

8. Serving Suggestions: Serve with tomato ketchup

9. Directions: & Cooking Tips: Peel and devein the shrimps

Nutrition: Calories: 193kcal, Fat: 13g, Carb: 1g, Proteins: 19g

Onion Pepper Shrimp

Preparation Time: 10 minutes

Cooking Time: 12 minutes

Servings: 4

Ingredients:

- 1 lb. shrimp, peeled, deveined, & tails removed
- 1/8 tsp cayenne pepper
- 1/2 tsp garlic powder
- 1 tsp chili powder
- 1 tbsp olive oil
- 1/2 onion, cut into 1-inch chunks
- 1 red bell pepper, cut into 1-inch chunks

Directions:

1. Add shrimp and remaining Ingredients into the mixing bowl and toss well.
2. Add shrimp mixture into the air fryer basket and cook at 330 F for 10-12 minutes. Shake air fryer basket halfway through.

Nutrition: Calories 183 Fat 5.6 g Carbohydrates 5.9 g Sugar 2.2 g Protein 26.4 g Cholesterol 239 mg

Old Bay Shrimp

Preparation Time:10 minutes

Cooking Time: 10 minutes

Servings:4

Ingredients:

- 12 oz shrimp, peeled
- oz pork rind, crushed
- 1 1/2 tsp old bay seasoning
- 1/4 cup mayonnaise

Directions:

1. In a shallow bowl, mix together crushed pork rind and old bay seasoning.
2. Add shrimp and mayonnaise into the mixing bowl and toss well.
3. Coat shrimp with pork rind mixture and place it into the air fryer basket.
4. Cook shrimp at 380 F for 10 minutes.

Nutrition: Calories 290 Fat 14.6 g Carbohydrates 4.8 g Sugar 0.9 g Protein 34.3 g Cholesterol 216 mg

Shrimp with Vegetables

Preparation Time:10 minutes

Cooking Time: 10 minutes

Servings:4

Ingredients:

- 1 lb. shrimp, peeled and deveined
- 1 tsp ginger, minced
- 1 tsp garlic, minced
- 2 tsp sesame oil
- 2 tbsp olive oil
- 4 tbsp soy sauce
- 1 lb. mushrooms, quartered
- 1 green bell pepper, sliced
- 1 lb. zucchini, cut into quarter-inch pieces

Directions:

1. Add shrimp and remaining Ingredients into the mixing bowl and toss well.
2. Add shrimp mixture into the air fryer basket and cook for 10 minutes. Shake basket halfway through.

Nutrition: Calories 278 Fat 11.8 g Carbohydrates 13.3 g Sugar 5.7 g Protein 32.1 g Cholesterol 239 mg

Delicious Buttery Shrimp

Preparation Time:10 minutes

Cooking Time: 6 minutes

Servings:4

Ingredients:

- 12 large shrimp, peeled and deveined
- 3 garlic cloves, minced
- 3 tbsp butter, melted

Directions:

1. In a bowl, add shrimp, garlic, butter, pepper, and salt and marinate shrimp for 15 minutes.
2. Remove shrimp from marinade and place into the air fryer basket and cook for 6 minutes.
3. Pour reserved marinade over shrimp and serve.

Nutrition: Calories 99 Fat 8.9 g Carbohydrates 1 g Sugar 0 g Protein 4 g Cholesterol 58 mg

Mexican Shrimp Fajitas

Preparation Time:10 minutes

Cooking Time: 8 minutes

Servings:4

Ingredients:

- 1 lb. jumbo shrimp, peeled and deveined
- 1 tsp chili powder
- 1 tsp paprika
- 1 oz fajita seasoning
- 2 garlic cloves, minced
- 1 tbsp olive oil
- 1 onion, sliced
- 1 yellow bell pepper, sliced
- 1 red bell pepper, sliced

Directions:

1. Add shrimp and remaining Ingredients into the large mixing bowl and toss well.
2. Add shrimp mixture into the air fryer basket and cook at 400 F for 8 minutes. Shake basket halfway through.

Nutrition: Calories 173 Fat 3.9 g Carbohydrates 13.6 g Sugar 6.3 g Protein 21.4 g Cholesterol 233 mg

Crisp & Juicy Cajun Shrimp

Preparation Time: 10 minutes

Cooking Time: 10 minutes

Servings: 4

Ingredients:

- 1 lb. shrimp, peeled and deveined
- 1 tbsp olive oil
- 1/2 tsp Cajun seasoning
- 1 garlic clove, minced

Directions:

1. Add shrimp, oil, Cajun seasoning, garlic, pepper, and salt into the mixing bowl. Toss well and place in the refrigerator for 1 hour.
2. Add shrimp mixture into the air fryer basket and cook at 350 F for 8-10 minutes. Turn halfway through.

Nutrition: Calories 166 Fat 5.4 g Carbohydrates 2 g Sugar 0 g Protein 25.9 g Cholesterol 239 mg

Lime Garlic Shrimp Kababs

Preparation Time:10 minutes

Cooking Time: 8 minutes

Servings:2

Ingredients:

- 1 cup raw shrimp
- 1 lime juice
- 1 garlic clove, minced

Directions:

1. Preheat the cosori air fryer to 350 F.
2. In a mixing bowl, mix together shrimp, lime juice, garlic, pepper, and salt.
3. Thread shrimp onto the skewers and place them into the air fryer basket and cook for 8 minutes. Turn halfway through.

Nutrition: Calories 201 Fat 2.8 g Carbohydrates 4.9 g Sugar 0.4 g Protein 37.2 g Cholesterol 342 mg

Tasty Chipotle Shrimp

Preparation Time:10 minutes

Cooking Time: 8 minutes

Servings:4

Ingredients:

- 1 1/2 lbs. shrimp, peeled and deveined
- 2 tbsp olive oil
- 4 tbsp lime juice
- 1 /4 tsp ground cumin
- 2 tsp chipotle in adobo

Directions:

1. Add shrimp, oil, lime juice, cumin, and chipotle in a zip-lock bag. Seal bag shake well and place it in the refrigerator for 30 minutes.
2. Thread marinated shrimp onto skewers and place skewers into the air fryer basket.
3. Cook at 350 F for 8 minutes.

Nutrition: Calories 274 Fat 10 g Carbohydrates 6.4 g Sugar 0.7 g Protein 39 g Cholesterol 359 mg

Tasty Shrimp Fajitas

Preparation Time: 10 minutes

Cooking Time: 22 minutes

Servings: 12

Ingredients:

- 1 lb. shrimp, tail-off
- 2 tbsp taco seasoning
- 1/2 cup onion, diced
- 1 green bell pepper, diced
- 1 red bell pepper, diced

Directions:

1. Spray air fryer basket with cooking spray.
2. Add shrimp, taco seasoning, onion, and bell peppers into the mixing bowl and toss well.
3. Place shrimp mixture into the air fryer basket and cook at 390 F for 12 minutes.
4. Stir shrimp mixture and cook for 10 minutes more.

Nutrition: Calories 55 Fat 0.8 g Carbohydrates 2.7 g Sugar 1.2 g Protein 9 g Cholesterol 80 mg

Easy Coconut Shrimp

Preparation Time:10 minutes

Cooking Time: 8 minutes

Servings:8

Ingredients:

- 2 eggs, lightly beaten
- 1 lb. large shrimp, peeled and deveined
- 1 cup unsweetened flaked coconut
- 1/4 cup coconut flour

Directions:

1. In a small bowl, add coconut flour.
2. In a shallow bowl, add eggs. In a separate shallow bowl, add flakes coconut.
3. Coat shrimp with coconut flour then dip in eggs and finally coat with flaked coconut.
4. Spray air fryer basket with cooking spray.
5. Place coated shrimp into the air fryer basket and cook at 400 F for 6-8 minutes. Turn shrimp halfway through.

Nutrition: Calories 112 Fat 4.8 g Carbohydrates 5.1 g Sugar 0.7 g Protein 12.9 g Cholesterol 122 mg

Shrimp & Vegetable Dinner

Preparation Time:10 minutes

Cooking Time: 10 minutes

Servings:4

Ingredients:

- 1 lb. jumbo shrimp, cleaned & peeled
- 2 tbsp olive oil
- 1 bell pepper, cut into 1-inch pieces
- 8 oz yellow squash, sliced into 1/4-inch half moons
- 1 medium zucchini, sliced into 1/4-inch half moons
- 6 oz sausage, cooked and sliced
- 1 tbsp Cajun seasoning
- 1/4 tsp kosher salt

Directions:

1. Add shrimp and remaining Ingredients into the large mixing bowl and toss well to coat.
2. Preheat the cosori air fryer to 400 F.
3. Add shrimp mixture into the air fryer basket and cook for 10 minutes. Shake air fryer basket 3 Times.

Nutrition: Calories 312 Fat 19.3 g Carbohydrates 5.8

g Sugar 5.4 g Protein 30.1 g Cholesterol 269 mg

Lemon Garlic Shrimp

Preparation Time: 10 minutes

Cooking Time: 15 minutes

Servings: 3

Ingredients:

- 1 lb. shrimp, peeled and deveined
- 1/4 tsp garlic powder
- 1 tbsp olive oil
- 1/2 fresh lemon
- 2 tbsp fresh parsley, chopped

Directions:

1. Toss shrimp with garlic powder, olive oil, pepper, and salt.
2. Add shrimp into the air fryer basket and cook at 400 F for 12-15 minutes. Shake basket halfway through.
3. Transfer shrimp to the serving bowl.
4. Squeeze lemon juice over shrimp.
5. Garnish with parsley and serve.

Nutrition: Calories 224 Fat 7.3 g Carbohydrates 3.6 g Sugar 0.3 g Protein 34.7 g Cholesterol 318 mg

Easy Cajun Shrimp

Preparation Time:10 minutes

Cooking Time: 6 minutes

Servings:2

Ingredients:

- 1/2 lb. shrimp, peeled and deveined
- 1 tbsp olive oil
- 1/4 tsp paprika
- 1/2 tsp old bay seasoning
- 1/2 tsp cayenne pepper
- Pinch of salt

Directions:

1. Preheat the cosori air fryer to 390 F.
2. Add shrimp and remaining Ingredients into the mixing bowl and toss well to coat.
3. Add shrimp into the air fryer basket and cook for 6 minutes.

Nutrition: Calories 197 Fat 9 g Carbohydrates 2.1 g Sugar 0.1 g Protein 25.9 g Cholesterol 239 mg

Sweet and Savory Breaded Shrimp

Preparation Time: 5 Minutes

Cooking Time: 20 Minutes

Servings: 2

Ingredients:

- 1/2 pound of fresh shrimp, peeled from their shells and rinsed
- 2 raw eggs
- 1/2 cup of breadcrumbs (we like Panko, but any brand or home recipe will do)
- 1/2 white onion, peeled and rinsed and finely chopped
- 1 teaspoon of ginger-garlic paste
- 1/2 teaspoon of turmeric powder
- 1/2 teaspoon of red chili powder
- 1/2 teaspoon of cumin powder
- 1/2 teaspoon of black pepper powder
- 1/2 teaspoon of dry mango powder
- Pinch of salt

Directions:

1. Preparing the ingredients. Cover the basket of the XL air fryer oven with a lining of tin

foil, leaving the edges uncovered to allow air to circulate through the basket.

2. Preheat the XL air fryer oven to 350 degrees.

3. In a mixing bowl, whisk the eggs until fluffy and until the yolks and whites are fully combined.

4. Dunk all the shrimp in the egg mixture, fully submerging.

5. In a separate mixing bowl, combine the bread crumbs with all the dry ingredients until evenly blended.

6. One by one, coat the egg-covered shrimp in the mixed dry Ingredients: so that fully covered, and place on the foil-lined air-fryer basket.

7. Air Frying. Set the air-fryer Timer to 20 minutes.

8. Halfway through the cooking Time, shake the handle of the air-fryer so that the breaded shrimp jostles inside and fry-coverage is even.

9. After 20 minutes, when the fryer shuts off, the shrimp will be perfectly cooked and

their breaded crust golden-brown and delicious! Using tongs, remove from the air fryer oven and set on a serving dish to cool.

Nutrition: Calories: 195; Fat: 11g; Protein: 25g; Sugar: 0g

Bacon Wrapped Shrimp

Preparation Time: 5 Minutes

Cooking Time: 5 Minutes

Servings: 4

Ingredients:

- 1¼ pound tiger shrimp, peeled and deveined
- 1-pound bacon

Directions:

1. Preparing the ingredients. With a slice of bacon, wrap each shrimp
2. Refrigerate for about 20 minutes.
3. Air Frying. Arrange the shrimp in the Oven rack/basket. Place the Rack on the middle-shelf of the XL air fryer oven. Cook for about 5-7 minutes.

Nutrition: Calories: 190; Fat: 11g; Protein: 21g; Sugar: 0g

Spicy Scallops

Preparation Time: 10 minutes

Cooking Time: 8 minutes

Servings: 4

Ingredients:

- 1 lb. scallops, thawed, washed, and pat dry with a paper towel
- 1 tsp garlic powder
- 1 tbsp chili powder
- 1 tbsp paprika
- 2 tbsp onion flakes
- Pepper
- Salt

Directions:

1. Spray air fryer basket with cooking spray.
2. In a mixing bowl, add scallops and remaining ingredients and toss well.
3. Add scallops into the air fryer basket and cook at 340 F for 8 minutes. Shake basket halfway through.
4. Serve and enjoy.

Nutrition: Calories 122 Fat 1.4 g Carbohydrates 7.3 g Sugar 1.4 g Protein 19.9 g Cholesterol 37 mg

Pesto Scallops

Preparation Time:10 minutes

Cooking Time: 8 minutes

Servings:4

Ingredients:

- 1 lb. sea scallops
- 2 tsp garlic, minced
- 3 tbsp heavy cream
- 1/4 cup basil pesto
- 1 tbsp olive oil
- Pepper
- Salt

Directions:

1. In a small pan, mix together oil, heavy cream, garlic, basil pesto, pepper, and salt, and simmer for 2-3 minutes.
2. Add scallops into the air fryer basket and cook at 320 F for 5 minutes.
3. Turn scallops and cook for 3 minutes more.
4. Transfer scallops into the mixing bowl. Pour sauce over the scallops and toss to coat.
5. Serve and enjoy.

Nutrition: Calories 171 Fat 8.5 g Carbohydrates 3.5

g Sugar 0 g Protein 19.4 g Cholesterol 53 mg

Old Bay Seasoned Crab Cakes

Preparation Time:10 minutes

Cooking Time: 10 minutes

Servings:5

Ingredients:

- 2 eggs
- 1/4 cup almond flour
- 2 tsp dried parsley
- 1 tbsp dried celery
- 1 tsp old bay seasoning
- 1 1/2 tbsp Dijon mustard
- 2 1/2 tbsp mayonnaise
- 18 oz can lump crab meat, drained
- 1/2 tsp salt

Directions:

1. Line air fryer basket with aluminum foil.
2. Add all Ingredients into the mixing bowl and mix until well combined. Place mixture in the refrigerator for 10 minutes.
3. Make five equal shapes of patties from mixture and place onto the aluminum foil in the air fryer basket.

4. Cook at 320 F for 10 minutes. Turn patties halfway through.

5. Serve and enjoy.

Nutrition: Calories 139 Fat 13.3 g Carbohydrates 4.2 g Sugar 0.7 g Protein 17.6 g Cholesterol 125 mg

Lemon Garlic Scallops

Preparation Time: 10 minutes

Cooking Time: 8 minutes

Servings: 4

Ingredients:

- 1 lb. sea scallops, pat dry with paper towels
- 1 tsp fresh thyme
- 1 garlic clove, minced
- 2 tbsp fresh lemon juice
- 1/4 cup olive oil
- Pepper
- Salt

Directions:

1. Season scallops with pepper and salt.
2. Spray air fryer basket with cooking spray.
3. Add scallops into the air fryer basket and cook at 400 F for 5-8 minutes or until the internal temperature of scallops reaches 120 F.
4. Transfer scallops to the serving bowl.
5. Heat olive oil in a pan on medium heat. Add garlic and sauté until garlic softens.

6. Add lemon juice and whisk until sauce is heated through.

7. Pour olive oil mixture overcooked scallops.

8. Garnish with thyme and serve.

Nutrition: Calories 212 Fat 13.5 g Carbohydrates 3.3 g Sugar 0.2 g Protein 19.2 g Cholesterol 37 mg

Lemon Caper Scallops

Preparation Time:10 minutes

Cooking Time: 6 minutes

Servings:2

Ingredients:

- 8 large sea scallops, clean and pat dry with a paper towel
- 1/2 tsp garlic, chopped
- 1 tsp lemon zest, grated
- 2 tsp capers, chopped
- 2 tbsp fresh parsley, chopped
- 1/4 cup olive oil
- Pepper
- Salt

Directions:

1. Season scallops with pepper and salt.
2. Spray air fryer basket with cooking spray.
3. Place scallops into the air fryer basket and cook at 400 F for 6 minutes or until the internal temperature of scallops reaches 120 F.

4. In a small bowl, mix together oil, garlic, lemon zest, capers, and parsley and drizzle over scallops and serve.

Nutrition: Calories 325 Fat 26.2 g Carbohydrates 3.7 g Sugar 0.1 g Protein 20.4 g Cholesterol 40 mg

Cajun Scallops

Preparation Time:10 minutes

Cooking Time: 6 minutes

Servings:1

Ingredients:

- 6 scallops, clean and pat dry with a paper towel
- 1/2 tsp Cajun seasoning
- Salt

Directions:

1. Preheat the cosori air fryer to 400 F.
2. Line air fryer basket with aluminum foil and spray with cooking spray.
3. Place scallops into the air fryer basket.
4. Season scallops with Cajun seasoning and salt and cooks for 6 minutes. Turn scallops halfway through.
5. Serve and enjoy.

Nutrition: Calories 158 Fat 1.4 g Carbohydrates 4.3 g Sugar 0 g Protein 30.2 g Cholesterol 59 mg

Flavorful Crab Cakes

Preparation Time: 10 minutes

Cooking Time: 10 minutes

Servings: 4

Ingredients:

- 8 oz lump crab
- 1 tsp old bay seasoning
- 1 tbsp Dijon mustard
- 2 tbsp almond flour
- 2 tbsp mayonnaise
- 2 tbsp green onion, chopped
- 1/4 cup bell pepper, chopped
- Pepper
- Salt

Directions:

1. Add lump crab and remaining Ingredients into the mixing bowl and mix until well combined.
2. Make four equal shapes of patties from mixture and place into the air fryer basket.
3. Spray top of patties with cooking spray.
4. Cook at 370 F for 10 minutes.
5. Serve and enjoy.

Nutrition: Calories 156 Fat 14.2 g Carbohydrates 6.7 g Sugar 1.5 g Protein 11.6 g Cholesterol 34 mg

Healthy Crab Cakes

Preparation Time:10 minutes

Cooking Time: 10 minutes

Servings:4

Ingredients:

- 8 oz lump crab meat
- 2 tbsp butter, melted
- 2 tsp Dijon mustard
- 1 tbsp mayonnaise
- 1 egg, lightly beaten
- 1/2 tsp old bay seasoning
- 1 green onion, sliced
- 2 tbsp parsley, chopped
- 1/4 cup almond flour
- Pepper
- Salt

Directions:

1. Add crab meat, mustard, mayonnaise, egg, old bay seasoning, green onion, parsley, almond flour, pepper, and salt into the mixing bowl and mix until well combined.

2. Make four equal shapes of patties from mixture and place on a waxed paper-lined dish and refrigerate for 30 minutes.
3. Brush melted butter over both sides of patties and place into the air fryer basket.
4. Cook patties at 350 F for 10 minutes. Turn halfway through.
5. Serve and enjoy.

Nutrition: Calories 136 Fat 13.7 g Carbohydrates 2.8 g Sugar 0.5 g Protein 10.3 g Cholesterol 89 mg

Crisp Bacon Wrapped Scallops

Preparation Time: 10 minutes

Cooking Time: 8 minutes

Servings: 4

Ingredients:

- 16 scallops, clean and pat dry with paper towels
- 8 bacon slices, cut each slice in half
- Pepper
- Salt

Directions:

1. Preheat the cosori air fryer to 400 F.
2. Place bacon slices into the air fryer basket and cook for 3 minutes. Turn halfway through.
3. Wrap each scallop in bacon slice and secure with a toothpick. Season with pepper and salt.
4. Spray wrapped scallops with cooking spray and place into the air fryer basket.
5. Cook scallops for 8 minutes. Turn halfway through.

6. Serve and enjoy.

Nutrition: Calories 311 Fat 16.8 g Carbohydrates 3.4 g Sugar 0 g Protein 34.2 g Cholesterol 81 mg

Soy and Ginger Shrimp

Preparation Time: 8 Minutes

Cooking Time: 10 Minutes

Servings: 4

Ingredients:

- 2 tablespoons olive oil
- 2 tablespoons scallions, finely chopped
- 2 cloves garlic, chopped
- 1 teaspoon fresh ginger, grated
- 1 tablespoon dry white wine
- 1 tablespoon balsamic vinegar
- 1/4 cup soy sauce
- 1 tablespoon sugar
- 1-pound shrimp
- Salt and ground black pepper, to taste

Directions:

1. Preparing the ingredients. To make the marinade, warm the oil in a saucepan; cook all ingredients, except the shrimp, salt, and black pepper. Now, let it cool.
2. Marinate the shrimp, covered, at least an hour, in the refrigerator.

3. Air Frying. After that, bake the shrimp at 350 degrees F for 8 to 10 minutes (depending on the size), turning once or twice. Season shrimp with salt and black pepper and serve right away.

Nutrition: Calories: 165 Carbs: 5.8 Fat: 4.5g Protein: 24g Fiber: 0g

Quick Paella

Preparation Time: 7 Minutes

Cooking Time: 15 Minutes

Servings: 4

Ingredients:

- 1 (10-ounce) package frozen cooked rice, thawed
- 1 (6-ounce) jar artichoke hearts, drained and chopped
- ¼ cup vegetable broth
- 1/2 teaspoon turmeric
- 1/2 teaspoon dried thyme
- 1 cup frozen cooked small shrimp
- 1/2 cup frozen baby peas
- 1 tomato, diced

Directions:

1. Preparing the ingredients. In a 6-by-6-by-2-inch pan, combine the rice, artichoke hearts, vegetable broth, turmeric, and thyme, and stir gently.
2. Air Frying. Place in the XL air fryer oven and bake for 8 to 9 minutes or until the rice is hot. Remove from the air fryer oven and

gently stir in the shrimp, peas, and tomato. Cook for 5 to 8 minutes or until the shrimp and peas are hot and the paella is bubbling.

Nutrition: Calories: 345 Fat: 1g Protein: 18g Fiber: 4g

Steamed Salmon and Sauce

Preparation Time: 5 minutes

Cooking Time: 10 minutes

Servings: 2

Ingredients:

- 1 cup Water
- x 6 oz Fresh Salmon
- Tsp Vegetable Oil
- A Pinch of Salt for Each Fish
- ½ cup Plain Greek Yogurt
- ½ cup Sour Cream
- Tbsp Finely Chopped Dill (Keep a bit for garnishing)
- A Pinch of Salt to Taste

Directions:

1. Pour the water into the tray of the air fryer oven and start heating to 285 degrees Fahrenheit.
2. Drizzle oil over the fish and spread it. Salt the fish to taste.
3. Now pop it into the air fryer oven for 10 min.

4. In the meantime, mix the yogurt, cream, dill and a bit of salt to make the sauce. When the fish is done, serve with the sauce and garnish with sprigs of dill.

Nutrition: Calories 185 Fat 11g Protein 21g Sugar 0g

Indian Fish Fingers

Preparation Time: 35 minutes

Cooking Time: 15 minutes

Servings: 4

Ingredients:

- 1/2-pound fish fillet
- 1 tablespoon finely chopped fresh mint leaves or any fresh herbs
- 1/3 cup bread crumbs
- 1 teaspoon ginger garlic paste or ginger and garlic powders
- 1 hot green chili finely chopped
- 1/2 teaspoon paprika
- Generous pinch of black pepper
- Salt to taste
- 3/4 tablespoons lemon juice
- 3/4 teaspoons garam masala powder
- 1/3 teaspoon rosemary
- 1 egg

Directions:

1. Start by removing any skin on the fish, washing, and patting dry. Cut the fish into fingers.

2. In a medium bowl mix together all ingredients except for fish, mint, and bread crumbs. Bury the fingers in the mixture and refrigerate for 30 minutes.

3. Remove from the bowl from the fridge and mix in mint leaves.

4. In a separate bowl beat the egg, pour bread crumbs into a third bowl. Dip the fingers in the egg bowl then toss them in the bread crumbs bowl.

5. Pour into the Oven rack/basket. Place the Rack on the middle-shelf of the Air fryer oven. Set temperature to 360 degrees Fahrenheit, and set Time to 15 minutes, toss the fingers halfway through.

Nutrition: Calories 187 Fat 7g Protein 11g Fiber 1g

Flying Fish

Preparation Time: 5 minutes

Cooking Time: 12 minutes

Servings: 6

Ingredients:

- Tbsp Oil
- 3–4 oz Breadcrumbs
- 1 Whisked Whole Egg in a Saucer/Soup Plate
- Fresh Fish Fillets
- Fresh Lemon (For serving)

Directions:

1. Preheat the air fryer to 350 degrees Fahrenheit. Mix the crumbs and oil until it looks nice and loose.
2. Dip the fish in the egg and coat lightly, then move on to the crumbs. Make sure the fillet is covered evenly.
3. Cook in the air fryer oven basket for roughly 12 minutes – depending on the size of the fillets you are using.
4. Serve with fresh lemon and chips to complete the duo.

Nutrition: Calories 480 Fat 37g Carbohydrates 9g Protein 49g

Pistachio-Crusted Lemon-Garlic Salmon

Preparation Time:5 minutes

Cooking Time: 20 minutes

Servings: 6

Ingredients :

- medium-sized salmon filets
- raw eggs
- ounces of melted butter
- 1 clove of garlic, peeled and finely minced
- 1 large-sized lemon
- 1 teaspoon of salt
- 1 tablespoon of parsley, rinsed, patted dry and chopped
- 1 teaspoon of dill, rinsed, patted dry and chopped
- ½ cup of pistachio nuts, shelled and coarsely crushed

Directions:

1. Cover the basket of the air fryer with a lining of tin foil, leaving the edges uncovered to allow air to circulate through the basket.

61

2. Preheat the air fryer oven to 350 degrees Fahrenheit.
3. In a mixing bowl, beat the eggs until fluffy and until the yolks and whites are fully combined.
4. Add the melted butter, the juice of the lemon, the minced garlic, the parsley and the dill to the beaten eggs, and stir thoroughly.
5. One by one, dunk the salmon filets into the wet mixture, then roll them in the crushed pistachios, coating completely.
6. Place the coated salmon fillets in the air fryer oven basket.
7. Set the air fryer oven Timer for 10 minutes.
8. When the air fryer shuts off, after 10 minutes, the salmon will be partly cooked and the crust beginning to crisp. Using tongs, turn each of the fish filets over.
9. Reset the air fryer oven to 350 degrees Fahrenheit for another 10 minutes.
10. After 10 minutes, when the air fryer shuts off, the salmon will be perfectly

cooked and the pistachio crust will be toasted and crispy. Using tongs, remove from the air fryer and serve.

Nutrition: Calories 185 Fat 11g Protein 21g Sugar 0g

Salmon Noodles

Preparation Time:5 minutes

Cooking Time: 16 minutes

Servings: 4

Ingredients:

- 1 Salmon Fillet
- 1 Tbsp Teriyaki Marinade
- ½ Ozs Soba Noodles, cooked and drained
- Ozs Firm Tofu
- Ozs Mixed Salad
- 1 Cup Broccoli
- Olive Oil
- Salt and Pepper to taste

Directions

1. Season the salmon with salt and pepper to taste, then coat with the teriyaki marinate. Set aside for 15 minutes

2. Preheat the air fryer oven at 350 degrees Fahrenheit, then cook the salmon for 8 minutes.

3. Whilst the air fryer is cooking the salmon, start slicing the tofu into small cubes.

4. Next, slice the broccoli into smaller chunks. Drizzle with olive oil.
5. Once the salmon is cooked, put the broccoli and tofu into the air fryer oven tray for 8 minutes.
6. Plate the salmon and broccoli tofu mixture over the soba noodles. Add the mixed salad to the side and serve.

Nutrition: Calories 185 Fat 11g Protein 21g Sugar 0g

Fried Calamari

Preparation Time: 8 minutes

Cooking Time: 7 minutes

Servings: 6-8

Ingredients:

- ½ tsp. salt
- ½ tsp. Old Bay seasoning
- 1/3 cup plain cornmeal
- ½ cup semolina flour
- ½ cup almond flour
- 5-6 cup olive oil
- 1 ½ pounds baby squid

Directions:

1. Rinse squid in cold water and slice tentacles, keeping just ¼-inch of the hood in one piece.
2. Combine 1-2 pinches of pepper, salt, Old Bay seasoning, cornmeal, and both flours together. Dredge squid pieces into flour mixture and place into the air fryer basket.

3. Spray liberally with olive oil. Cook 15 minutes at 345 degrees Fahrenheit till coating turns a golden brown.

Nutrition: Calories 211 Carbohydrates 55g Fat 6g Protein 21g

Mustard-Crusted Fish Fillets

Preparation Time: 5 minutes

Cooking Time: 8 to 11 minutes

Servings: 4

Ingredients:

- teaspoons low-sodium yellow mustard
- 1 tablespoon freshly squeezed lemon juice
- (3.5-ounce) sole fillets
- ½ teaspoon dried thyme
- ½ teaspoon dried marjoram
- 1/8 teaspoon freshly ground black pepper
- 1 slice low-sodium whole-wheat bread, crumbled
- teaspoons olive oil

Directions:

1. 1 In a small bowl, mix the mustard and lemon juice. Spread this evenly over the fillets. Place them in the air fryer basket.
2. In another small bowl, mix the thyme, marjoram, pepper, bread crumbs, and olive oil. Mix until combined.

3. Gently but firmly press the spice mixture onto the top of each fish fillet.

4. Bake for 8 to 11 minutes at 320 degrees Fahrenheit, or until the fish reaches an internal temperature of at least 145 degrees Fahrenheit on a meat thermometer and the topping is browned and crisp. Serve immediately.

Nutrition: Calories 142 Fat 4g Saturated Fat 1g Protein 20g Carbohydrates 5g Sodium 140g Fiber 1g Sugar 1g

Fish and Vegetable Tacos

Preparation Time:15 minutes

Cooking Time: 9 to 12 minutes

Servings: 4

Ingredients:

- 1-pound white fish fillets, such as sole or co
- teaspoons olive oil
- tablespoons freshly squeezed lemon juice, divided
- 1 1/2cups chopped red cabbage
- 1 large carrot, grated
- 1/2cup low-sodium salsa
- 1/3 cup low-fat Greek yogurt
- soft low-sodium whole-wheat tortillas

Directions:

1. 1 Brush the fish with the olive oil and sprinkle with 1 -tablespoon of lemon juice. Air-fry in the air fryer basket for 9 to 12 minutes at 390 degrees Fahrenheit, or until the fish just flakes when tested with a fork.
2. Meanwhile, in a medium bowl, stir together the remaining 2 tablespoons of lemon juice, the red cabbage, carrot, salsa, and yogurt.

3. When the fish is cooked, remove it from the air fryer basket and break it up into large pieces.

4. Offer the fish, tortillas, and the cabbage mixture, and let each person assemble a taco.

Nutrition: Calories 209 Fat 3g Saturated Fat 0g Protein 18g Carbohydrates 30g Sodium 116g Fiber 1g Sugar 4g

Lighter Fish and Chips

Preparation Time:10 minutes

Cooking Time: 11 to 15 minutes (chips); 10 to 14 minutes (cod fillets)

Servings: 4

Ingredients:

- russet potatoes, peeled, thinly sliced, rinsed, and patted dry
- 1egg white
- 1 tablespoon freshly squeezed lemon juice
- 1/3 cup ground almonds
- slices low-sodium whole-wheat bread, finely crumbled
- 1/2 teaspoon dried basil
- (4-ounce) cod fillets

Directions:

1. 1 Preheat the oven to warm.
2. Put the potato slices in the air fryer basket and air-fry for 11 to 15 minutes at 390 degrees Fahrenheit, or until crisp and brown. With tongs, turn the fries twice during cooking.

3. Meanwhile, in a shallow bowl, beat the egg white and lemon juice until frothy.

4. On a plate, mix the almonds, bread crumbs, and basil.

5. One at a Time, dip the fillets into the egg white mixture and then into the almond–bread crumb mixture to coat. Place the coated fillets on a wire rack to dry while the fries cook.

6. When the potatoes are done, transfer them to a baking sheet and keep warm in the oven on low heat.

7. Air-fry the fish in the air fryer basket for 10 to 14 minutes, or until the fish reaches an internal temperature of at least 140 degrees Fahrenheit on a meat thermometer and the coating is browned and crisp. Serve immediately with the potatoes.

Nutrition: Calories 247 Fat 5g Saturated Fat 0g Protein 27g Carbohydrates 25g Sodium 131g Fiber 3g Sugar 3g

Snapper with Fruit

Preparation Time:15 minutes

Cooking Time: 9 to 13 minutes

Servings: 4

Ingredients:

- (4-ounce) red snapper fillets
- teaspoons olive oil
- nectarines, halved and pitted
- plums, halved and pitted
- 1 cup red grapes
- 1 tablespoon freshly squeezed lemon juice
- 1 tablespoon honey
- ½ teaspoon dried thyme

Directions:

1. 1 Put the red snapper in the air fryer basket and drizzle with the olive oil. Air-fry for 4 minutes at 390 degrees Fahrenheit.
2. Remove the basket and add the nectarines and plums. Scatter the grapes over all.
3. Drizzle with the lemon juice and honey and sprinkle with the thyme.
4. Return the basket to the air fryer and air-fry for 5 to 9 minutes more, or until the fish

flakes when tested with a fork and the fruit is tender. Serve immediately.

Nutrition: Calories 245 Fat 4g Saturated Fat 1g Protein 25g Carbohydrates 28g Sodium 73g Fiber 3g Sugar 24g

Tuna Wraps

Preparation Time:10 minutes

Cooking Time: 4 to 7 minutes

Servings: 4

Ingredients:

- 1-pound fresh tuna steak, cut into 1-inch cubes
- 1 tablespoon grated fresh ginger
- garlic cloves, minced
- ½ teaspoon toasted sesame oil
- low-sodium whole-wheat tortillas
- ¼ cup low-fat mayonnaise
- cups shredded romaine lettuce
- 1 red bell pepper, thinly sliced

Directions:

1. 1 In a medium bowl, mix the tuna, ginger, garlic, and sesame oil. Let it stand for 10 minutes.
2. Grill the tuna in the air fryer for 4 to 7 minutes at 390 degrees Fahrenheit, or until done to your liking and lightly browned.

3. Make wraps with the tuna, tortillas, mayonnaise, lettuce, and bell pepper. Serve immediately.

Nutrition: Calories 288 Fat 7g Saturated Fat 2g Protein 31g Carbohydrates 26g Sodium 135g Fiber 1g Sugar 1g

Tuna and Fruit Kebabs

Preparation Time:15 minutes

Cooking Time: 8 to 12 minutes

Servings: 4

Ingredients:

- 1 pound tuna steaks, cut into 1-inch cubes
- ½ cup canned pineapple chunks, drained, juice reserved
- ½ cup large red grapes
- 1 tablespoon honey
- teaspoons grated fresh ginger
- 1 teaspoon olive oil
- Pinch cayenne pepper

Directions:

1. 1 Thread the tuna, pineapple, and grapes on 8 bamboo or 4 metal skewers that fit in the air fryer.
2. In a small bowl, whisk the honey, 1 tablespoon of reserved pineapple juice, the ginger, olive oil, and cayenne. Brush this mixture over the kebabs. Let them stand for 10 minutes.

3. Grill the kebabs for 8 to 12 minutes at 370 degrees Fahrenheit, or until the tuna reaches an internal temperature of at least 145 degrees Fahrenheit on a meat thermometer, and the fruit is tender and glazed, brushing once with the remaining sauce. Discard any remaining marinade. Serve immediately.

Nutrition: Calories 181 Fat 2g Saturated Fat 0g Protein 18g Carbohydrates 13g Sodium 43g Fiber 1g Sugar 12g

Asian Swordfish

Preparation Time:10 minutes

Cooking Time: 6 to 11 minutes

Servings: 4

Ingredients:

- (4-ounce) swordfish steaks
- ½ teaspoon toasted sesame oil
- 1 jalapeño pepper, finely minced
- garlic cloves, grated
- 1 tablespoon grated fresh ginger
- ½ teaspoon Chinese five-spice powder
- 1/8 teaspoon freshly ground black pepper
- tablespoons freshly squeezed lemon juice

Directions:

1. 1 Place the swordfish steaks on a work surface and drizzle with the sesame oil.
2. In a small bowl, mix the jalapeño, garlic, ginger, five-spice powder, pepper, and lemon juice. Rub this mixture into the fish and let it stand for 10 minutes.
3. Roast the swordfish in the air fryer for 6 to 11 minutes at 380 degrees Fahrenheit, or until the swordfish reaches an internal

temperature of at least 140 degrees Fahrenheit on a meat thermometer. Serve immediately.

Nutrition: Calories 187 Fat 6g Saturated Fat 1g Protein 29g Carbohydrates 2g Sodium 132g Fiber 0g Sugar 1g

Salmon Spring Rolls

Preparation Time: 20 minutes

Cooking Time: 8 to 10 minutes

Servings: 4

Ingredients:

- ½ pound salmon fillet
- 1 teaspoon toasted sesame oil
- 1 onion, sliced
- rice paper wrappers
- 1 yellow bell pepper, thinly sliced
- 1 carrot, shredded
- 1/3 cup chopped fresh flat-leaf parsley
- ¼ cup chopped fresh basil

Directions:

1. 1 Put the salmon in the air fryer basket and drizzle with the sesame oil. Add the onion. Air-fry for 8 to 10 minutes, or until the salmon just flakes when tested with a fork and the onion is tender.
2. Meanwhile, fill a small shallow bowl with warm water. One at a Time, dip the rice paper wrappers into the water and place on a work surface.

3. Top each wrapper with one-eighth each of the salmon and onion mixture, yellow bell pepper, carrot, parsley, and basil. Roll up the wrapper, folding in the sides, to enclose the ingredients.

4. If you like, bake in the air fryer at 380 degrees Fahrenheit for 7 to 9 -minutes, until the rolls are crunchy. Cut the rolls in half to serve.

Nutrition: Calories 95 Fat 2g Saturated Fat 0g Protein 13g Carbohydrates 8g Sodium 98g Fiber 2g Sugar 2g

Salmon on Bed of Fennel and Carrot

Preparation Time: 15 minutes

Cooking Time: 13 to 14 minutes

Servings: 4

Ingredients:

- 1 fennel bulb, thinly sliced
- 1 large carrot, peeled and sliced
- 1 small onion, thinly sliced
- ¼ cup low-fat sour cream
- ¼ teaspoon coarsely ground pepper
- (5 ounce) salmon fillets

Directions:

1. 1 Combine the fennel, carrot, and onion in a bowl and toss.
2. Put the vegetable mixture into a 6-inch metal pan. Roast in the air fryer for 4 minutes at 400 degrees Fahrenheit or until the vegetables are crisp tender.
3. Remove the pan from the air fryer. Stir in the sour cream and sprinkle the vegetables with the pepper.
4. Top with the salmon fillets.

5. Return the pan to the air fryer. Roast for another 9 to 10 minutes or until the salmon just barely flakes when tested with a fork.

Nutrition: Calories 253 Fat 9g Saturated Fat 1g Protein 31g Carbohydrates 12g Sodium 115g Fiber 3g Sugar 5g

Scallops with Green Vegetables

Preparation Time:15 minutes

Cooking Time: 8 to 11 minutes

Servings: 4

Ingredients:

- 1 cup green beans
- 1 cup frozen peas
- 1 cup frozen chopped broccoli
- teaspoons olive oil
- ½ teaspoon dried basil
- ½ teaspoon dried oregano
- ounces sea scallops

Directions:

1. 1 In a large bowl, toss the green beans, peas, and broccoli with the olive oil. Place in the air fryer basket. Air-fry for 4 to 6 minutes, or until the vegetables are crisp-tender.
2. Remove the vegetables from the air fryer basket and sprinkle with the herbs. Set aside.

3. In the air fryer basket, put the scallops and air-fry for 4 to 5 minutes at 400 degrees Fahrenheit, or until the scallops are firm and reach an internal temperature of just 145 degrees Fahrenheit on a meat thermometer.

4. Toss scallops with the vegetables and serve immediately.

Nutrition: Calories 124 Fat 3g Saturated Fat 0g Protein 14g Carbohydrates 11g Sodium 56g Fiber 3g Sugar 5g

Ranch Flavored Tilapia

Preparation Time:15 minutes

Cooking Time: 13 minutes

Servings: 4

Ingredients:

- ¾ cup cornflakes, crushed
- 1-ounce dry ranch mix
- and ½ tablespoons vegetable oil
- whole eggs
- pieces 6 ounces each tilapia fillets

Directions:

1. Take a shallow bowl, crack in eggs and beat them well
2. Take another bowl and add cornflakes, ranch dressing
3. oil and mix well until you have a crumbly ix
4. Dip fish fillets into the egg
5. coat well with bread crumbs mixture
6. Press "Power Button" on your Air Fryer and select "Air Fry" mode
7. Press the Time Button and set Time to 13 minutes

8. Push Temp Button and set temp to 356 degrees F

9. Press the "Start/Pause" button and start the device

10. Once the appliance beeps to indicated that it is pre-heated, arrange tilapia into Air Fryer basket, insert into oven

11. Let it cook until done, serve, and enjoy!

Nutrition: Calories: 267 Fat: 12 g Saturated Fat: 3 g Carbohydrates: 5 g Fiber: 0.2 g Sodium: 168 mg Protein: 34 g

Butter Up Salmon

Preparation Time: 10 minutes

Cooking Time: 10 minutes

Servings: 2

Ingredients:

- pieces 6 ounces salmon fillets
- Salt and pepper to taste
- tablespoon butter, melted

Directions:

1. Season salmon fillet well with salt and pepper, coat them with butter
2. Press "Power Button" on your Air Fryer and select "Air Fry" mode
3. Press the Time Button and set Time to 20 minutes
4. Push Temp Button and set temp to 320 degrees F
5. Press the "Start/Pause" button and start the device
6. Once the appliance beeps to indicated that it is pre-heated, transfer fillets to a greased Air Fryer basket and push into oven
7. Serve and enjoy!

Nutrition: Calories: 270 Fat: 16 g Saturated Fat: 5.2 g Carbohydrates: 0 g Fiber: 0 g Sodium: 193 mg Protein: 33 g

Lemon Salmon

Preparation Time: 10 minutes

Cooking Time: 8 minutes

Servings: 3

Ingredients:

- and ½ pounds salmon
- ½ teaspoon red chili powder
- Salt and pepper to taste
- 1 lemon, cut into slices
- 1 tablespoon fresh dill, chopped

Directions:

1. Season salmon with chili powder, salt, pepper generously
2. Press "Power Button" on your Air Fryer and select "Air Fry" mode
3. Press the Time Button and set Time to 8 minutes
4. Push Temp Button and set temp to 375 degrees F
5. Press the "Start/Pause" button and start the device

6. Once the appliance beeps to indicated that it is pre-heated, arrange salmon fillets in the Air Fryer cooking basket
7. Push into Air Fryer Oven and cook until the Timer runs out
8. Garnish with fresh dill and serve hot!

Nutrition: Calories: 305 Fat: 14 g Saturated Fat: 2 g Carbohydrates: 1.3 g Fiber: 0.4 g Sodium: 156 mg Protein: 44 g

Hearty Spiced Salmon

Preparation Time: 10 minutes

Cooking Time: 11 minutes

Servings: 2

Ingredients:

- teaspoon smoked paprika
- 1 teaspoon cayenne pepper
- 1 teaspoon onion powder
- 1 teaspoon garlic powder
- Salt and pepper to taste
- pieces 6 ounces salmon fillets
- teaspoons olive oil

Directions:

1. Take a small bowl and add spices, mix them well
2. Drizzle salmon fillets with oil, rub the fillets with spice mixture
3. Press "Power Button" on your Air Fryer and select "Air Fry" mode
4. Press the Time Button and set Time to 11 minutes
5. Push Temp Button and set temp to 390 degrees F

6. Press the "Start/Pause" button and start the device

7. Once the appliance beeps to indicated that it is pre-heated, arrange salmon fillets in the Air Fryer cooking basket

8. Push into Air Fryer Oven and cook until the Timer runs out

9. Serve and enjoy!

Nutrition: Calories: 280 Fat: 15 g Saturated Fat: 2 g Carbohydrates: 3 g Fiber: 1 g Sodium: 0.8 mg Protein: 33 g

Cajun Shrimp

Preparation Time: 10 minutes

Cooking Time: 7 minutes

Servings: 4

Ingredients:

- and ¼ pound tiger shrimp, about 16-20 pieces
- ¼ teaspoon cayenne pepper
- ½ teaspoon old bay seasoning
- ¼ teaspoon smoked paprika
- 1 pinch of salt
- 1 tablespoon olive oil

Directions:

1. Preheat your Air Fryer to 390 degrees F in "AIR FRY" mode
2. Take a mixing bowl and add Ingredients:(except shrimp), mix well
3. Dip the shrimp into spice mixture and oil
4. Transfer the shrimp to your cooking basket and cook for 5 minutes
5. Serve and enjoy!

Nutrition: Calories: 180 Fat: 2 g Saturated Fat: 1 g Carbohydrates: 5 g Fiber: 0 g Sodium: 970 mg

Protein: 23 g

Air Fried Dragon Shrimp

Preparation Time:10 minutes

Cooking Time: 10 minutes

Servings: 4

Ingredients:

- 1-pound raw shrimp, peeled and deveined
- A ½ cup of soy sauce
- eggs
- tablespoons olive oil
- cup yellow onion, diced
- ¼ cup flour
- ½ teaspoon red pepper, ground
- ½ teaspoon ginger, grounded

Directions:

1. Preheat your air fryer to 350 degrees F in "AIR FRY" mode
2. Add all the ingredients except for the shrimp to make the batter
3. Set it aside for 10 minutes
4. Dip each shrimp into the batter to coat all sides
5. Place them on the air fryer basket
6. Cook for 10 minutes

7. Serve and enjoy!

Nutrition: Calories: 600 Fat: 6 g Saturated Fat: 2 g
Carbohydrates: 59 g Fiber: 8 g Sodium: 690 mg
Protein: 31 g

Mushroom and Tilapia

Preparation Time: 10 minutes

Cooking Time: 16 minutes

Servings: 4

Ingredients:

- ½ cup yellow onion, sliced thin
- ounces filets tilapia
- tablespoons olive oil
- cups mushroom, sliced
- tablespoons soy sauce
- cloves garlic, minced
- tablespoon honey
- tablespoons rice vinegar
- and ½ teaspoon salt
- 1 tablespoon red chili flakes

Directions:

1. Preheat your air fryer to 350 degrees F in "AIR FRY" mode
2. Season the fish with half the salt
3. Drizzle with half the oil
4. Cook for 15 minutes
5. Take a large skillet and add remaining oil and heat it

6. Add the onion, garlic, and mushroom when it is hot
7. Cook until onions are soft
8. Stir in the soy sauce, honey, vinegar, and chili flakes
9. Simmer for 1 minute
10. Serve with mushroom sauce and enjoy!

Nutrition: Calories: 300 Fat: 10 g Saturated Fat: 2 g Carbohydrates: 12 g Fiber: 4 g Sodium: 609 mg Protein: 45 g

Fish Tacos

Preparation Time:10 Minutes

Cooking Time: 9 Minutes

Servings: 4

Ingredients:

- cod fillets, cut into 1-inch cubes
- Salt and black pepper to taste
- ½ lime, juiced
- ½ cup all-purpose flour
- large egg
- lightly beaten
- 1 cup panko breadcrumbs
- Olive oil for brushing
- medium corn tortillas
- ½ cup shredded red cabbage
- 1 medium avocado, pitted, peeled, and chopped
- tbsp chopped fresh cilantro
- 1 cup sour cream
- Lime wedges for serving

Directions:

1. Insert the dripping pan in the bottom part of the air fryer and preheat the oven at Air

Fry mode at 400 F for 2 to 3 minutes. Lightly brush the rotisserie basket with some olive oil and set aside.

2. Season the fish with salt, black pepper, and lime juice.

3. Pour the flour onto a plate and the breadcrumbs onto another. Dredge the fish pieces lightly on the flour, then in the eggs, and the breadcrumbs. Put the coated fish in the rotisserie basket and fit into the oven using the rotisserie lift.

4. Set the Timer for 9 minutes or until the fish pieces are golden brown.

5. To serve, lay the tortillas individually on a clean, flat surface and add the fish pieces. Top with the cabbage, avocado, cilantro, sour cream, and lime wedges.

6. Serve immediately.

Nutrition: Calories 275 Total Fat 11.34g Total Carbs 19.39g Fiber 25g Protein 23.37g Sugar 1.5g Sodium 422mg

Asian Coconut Shrimp

Preparation Time: 10 minutes

Cooking Time: 8 minutes

Servings: 4

Ingredients:

- ½ cup all-purpose flour
- large eggs
- 2/3 cup unsweetened coconut flakes
- 1/3 cup panko breadcrumbs
- 24 medium shrimps
- Salt and black pepper to taste
- Olive oil

Directions:

1. Insert the dripping pan in the bottom part of the air fryer and preheat the oven at Air Fry mode at 400 F for 2 to 3 minutes. Lightly brush the rotisserie basket with some olive oil and set aside.

2. Pour the flour into a shallow plate, whisk the eggs in a bowl, and mix the coconut flakes with breadcrumbs on another plate.

3. Season the shrimps with salt, black pepper, and dredge lightly in the flour. Proceed to coat in the eggs and then, generously, in the breadcrumb's mixture.
4. Spray the coated shrimps with some olive oil and arrange it in the rotisserie basket. Fit the basket in the oven using the rotisserie lift and set the Timer for 8 minutes or until the shrimps are golden brown.
5. When ready, transfer the shrimps to serving plates and serve warm with sweet coconut dipping sauce.

Nutrition: Calories 190 Total Fat 7.16g Total Carbs 20.88g Fiber 2g Protein 10.32g Sugar 5.95g Sodium 281mg

Mahi Fahrenheit with Herby Buttery Drizzle

Preparation Time: 10 minutes

Cooking Time: 12 minutes

Servings: 4

Ingredients:

- (6 oz) Mahi Fahrenheit fillets
- Salt and black pepper to taste
- Olive oil for spraying
- 2/3 cup butter, melted
- tbsp chopped fresh parsley
- ½ tbsp chopped fresh dill

Directions:

1. Insert the dripping pan in the bottom part of the air fryer and preheat the oven at Bake mode at 400 F for 2 to 3 minutes.
2. Season the Mahi Fahrenheit fillets with salt, black pepper, and grease lightly with some olive oil. Lay the fish on the cooking tray and fit onto the middle rack of the oven.
3. Close the lid and set the Timer for 12 minutes.

4. Once the fish cooks, transfer to a serving platter. Whisk the butter with the parsley and dill, and drizzle the mixture on the fish before serving.

5. Enjoy immediately.

Nutrition: Calories 529 Total Fat 46.54g Total Carbs 9.25g Fiber 5.6g Protein 20.26g Sugar 1.28g Sodium 422mg

Classic Lemon Pepper Haddock

Preparation Time: 10 minutes

Cooking Time: 12 minutes

Servings: 4

Ingredients:

- ¼ cup all-purpose flour
- egg whites
- 1/3 cup panko breadcrumbs
- tsp lemon pepper
- egg whites
- (8 oz) haddock fillets
- Salt to taste
- slices lemon
- Chopped parsley to garnish

Directions:

1. Insert the dripping pan in the bottom part of the air fryer and preheat the oven at Air Fry mode at 400 F for 2 to 3 minutes.
2. Pour the flour in a shallow plate, mix the breadcrumbs and lemon peppers in another shallow dish, whisk the egg whites lightly in

a medium bowl, and season the fish lightly with salt.

3. Dredge the fish lightly in the flour, then coat in the egg whites, and then generously in the breadcrumb's mixture.

4. Lay the fish on the cooking tray, grease lightly with cooking spray, and fit onto the middle rack of the oven. Close the air fryer and set the Timer for 12 minutes.

5. Once the fish cooks, transfer to a serving platter and serve immediately with the lemon and parsley garnish.

Nutrition: Calories 208 Total Fat 1.22g Total Carbs 10.95g Fiber 1.1g Protein 36.88g Sugar 2.14g Sodium 476mg

www.ingramcontent.com/pod-product-compliance
Lightning Source LLC
Chambersburg PA
CBHW071112030426
42336CB00013BA/2044